Anchal Goel
Bareera Iram
Akash Bhatnagar

OZONE: UNVEILING THE BOON IN PEDIATRIC DENTISTRY

Anchal Goel
Bareera Iram
Akash Bhatnagar

OZONE: UNVEILING THE BOON IN PEDIATRIC DENTISTRY

LAP LAMBERT Academic Publishing

Cover image: www.ingimage.com

Publisher:
LAP LAMBERT Academic Publishing
is a trademark of
Dodo Books Indian Ocean Ltd. and OmniScriptum S.R.L publishing group

120 High Road, East Finchley, London, N2 9ED, United Kingdom
Str. Armeneasca 28/1, office 1, Chisinau MD-2012, Republic of Moldova, Europe
Managing Directors: Ieva Konstantinova, Victoria Ursu
info@omniscriptum.com

Printed at: see last page
ISBN: 978-620-8-44479-2

OZONE: UNVEILING THE BOON IN PEDIATRIC DENTISTRY

ACKNOWLEDGEMENT

For the culmination of this Library Dissertation, I have been guided and assisted by many people in their own way. I hereby take this opportunity to pay my gratitude and sincere thanks to all those who have helped me for its completion.

First, I would like to thank Almighty GOD and my beloved BANKEY for bestowing countless blessings upon me.

I am grateful to respected **Dr. Manish Goyal**, Principal, Teerthanker Mahaveer Dental College and Research Centre, Moradabad for his constant support and for being a source of tremendous inspiration.

I would like to thank **Dr. Sandeep A. Bailwad,** Professor & Head, Department of Pedodontics and Preventive Dentistry, Teerthanker Mahaveer Dental College and Research Centre, for their outstanding teaching, support and guidance and help all throughout.

I am at loss of words to express my gratitude to my guiding light **Dr. Akash Bhatnagar** Reader, as this work is a direct extension of his guidance, knowledge and wisdom bestowed upon me. I am deeply indebted for his complete support, affectionate and constructive criticism throughout the time of this dissertation. It is due to his feeling for detail and accuracy and constant motivation that I have been able to complete my dissertation in the stipulated time period.

I also thank respected **Dr. Kapil Dev Gupta,** Professor; **Dr. Zakiya Perveen**, Senior Lecturer; **Dr. Urvashi Bala**, Senior Lecturer; Department of Pedodontics and Preventive Dentistry, Teerthanker Mahaveer Dental College and Research Centre,

Moradabad who has provided me extensive personal and professional guidance and for providing me with the ideal academic environment for completing my dissertation.

I also take this opportunity to thank my seniors **Dr. Medha Roy, Dr. Sushma Singh, Dr. Zainab Khan, Dr. Manan Phalke** and **Dr. Aarti Yadav** for their unflinching support and constant encouragement.

I also thank My batch mates **Dr. Saman Seraj, Dr. Palak Mishra, Dr. Bareera Iram** and **Dr. Aatya Takuli** who had also helped me in compiling the enormous data of the study, and I thank them for their friendship, love, and unyielding support.

Words would not be sufficient to express my deep sense of gratitude to my parents for their unwavering and unconditional support. A special thanks to my Father **Dr. Ravinder Goel** and my Mother **Mrs. Seema Goel** and my sibling **Dr Nancy Goel Sparsh Goel and Bunny** for being a source of tremendous support and comfort to me at all times. I extend my warmest thanks to **Dr. Sajal Agarwal** who has provided me extensive personal and professional guidance.

Dr. Anchal Goel

CONTENTS

Introduction

INTRODUCTION

What it is and what does it do?

- Ozone is a chemical compound consisting of three atoms of oxygen. Ozone protects living organism by surrounding the earth at an altitude of 50,000 to 100,000 feet. Its molecular weight is 47, 98 g/mol and thermodynamically highly instable compound that, dependent on system conditions like temperature and pressure, decompose to pure oxygen with a short half-life. Ozone is 1.6-fold denser and 10-fold more soluble in water (49.0 mL in 100 mL water at 0° C) than oxygen.[1]
- Ozone is an unstable gas that cannot be stored and should be used at once because it has a half-life of 40 min at 20 °C.
- Ozone also known as trioxygen is an allotropic form of oxygen and an unstable gas which occur naturally by the action of ultraviolet rays on oxygen in the outer atmosphere. [2]The ozone layer absorbs the sun's harmful ultraviolet rays, thus allowing for survival of plant and animal life.[1]
- Ozone is a powerful oxidizer, it kills bacteria, fungi, viruses, protozoa and parasites.[3]
- Ozone has antimicrobial, ant-inflammatory, immuno-modulating, biosynthetic, bioenergetic, antihypoxic, analgesic and hemostatic effects.[4]
- The antibacterial effect of ozone is based on the inhibition of their metabolic activity and the lysis of bacterial cell wall.[5]
- The main antiviral actions of ozone are the change of the capsid and the irreversible destruction of viral DNA.[5]

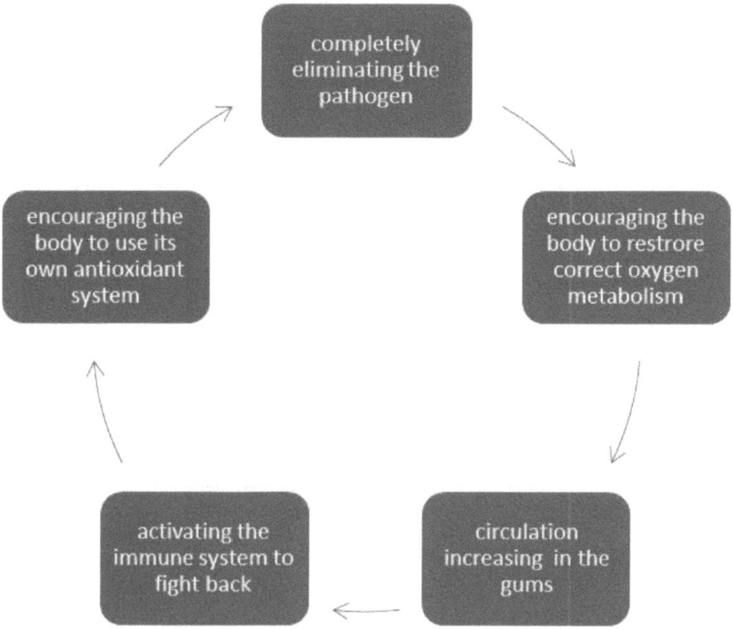
completely eliminating the pathogen
encouraging the body to restrore correct oxygen metabolism
circulation increasing in the gums
activating the immune system to fight back
encouraging the body to use its own antioxidant system

HISTORY

- Father of ozone therapy German chemist **Christian Friedrich Schonbein** of the University of Basel in Switzerland. In 1840, he discovered is a powerful oxidizer, it helps to clean atmosphere from harmful compounds. ozone when electric discharge passed through water; a strange smell was emanated, which he terms ozone. [6]

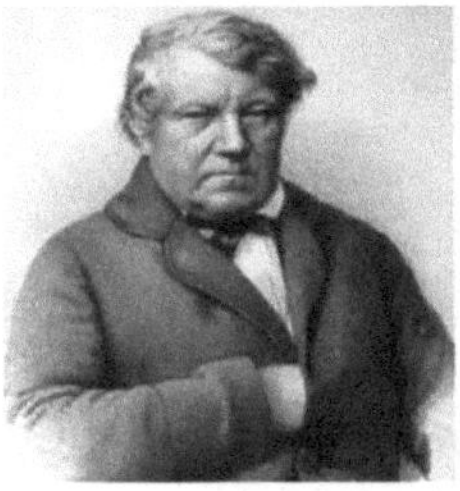

○

- **1857– Joachim Hensler**, a German physicist and **Hanswolf** German Physician developed first ozone generator for medical use.[6]
- **1870- D. C. Lender**, the first used ozone in medical field for purifying blood in test tubes.[6]
- **1930- A German Dentist**, Dr. E. A. use ozone in regular basis in his dental.[7]
- **1957- Werner Von Siemens** in Germany developed first ozone generator.[6]
- In the early 20th century, the Food and Drug act revised its uses and effects in the field of medicine.
- **1950- Dr. E. A. fish and Dr Ernst Payr**, the regular use of ozone in dentistry was first started further extended its application for general surgery.[6]
- **2001**- the beginning of dental application research was started with the approval of an (Institutional Review Board for Human Research) for human research from capital university of integrative medicine in Washington.[7]

- **2001- Dr. Sieg Fried** wrote a textbook about use of ozone in medicine.[7]
- **2001**- The first formal lecture on oxygen / ozone therapy was done at capital university.[6]
- **2004- Prof. Edward Lyrich** published 'Ozone – the revolution in dentistry.[7]

Review of Literature

REVIEW OF THE LITERATURE

Ebensberger et al.[8] in this year 2002 to evaluate the effect of irrigation with ozonated water on the proliferation of cells in the periodontal ligament adhering to the root surfaces. The teeth were randomly treated by intensive irrigation with ozonated water for 2 min or irrigation with a sterile isotonic saline solution, serving as a control group The periodontal cells of these teeth were studied immunohistochemically to mark proliferating cell nuclear antigen (PCNA). Two-minute irrigation of the avulsed teeth with non-isotonic ozonated water might lead not only to a mechanical cleansing, but also decontaminate the root surface, with no negative effect on periodontal cells remaining on the tooth surface.

Murakami et al.[9] in this year 2002 to examine the bactericidal and virucidal effectiveness of a denture cleaner that uses ozone. Bactericidal and virucidal effectiveness of 10 ppm ozone (as an effective chemical of a commercial denture cleaner) against methicillin-resistant S. aureus and T1 phage. The use of ozone in this denture cleaner is effective against methicillin-resistant S. aureus and viruses.

Nagayoshi et al.[10] in this year 2004 to examine the effect of ozonated water on oral microorganisms and dental plaque. Dental plaque samples were treated with 4 mL of ozonated water for 10 s. They came to the conclusion that ozonated water was effective for killing gram positive and gram-negative oral microorganisms and oral candida albicans in pure culture as well as bacteria in plaque biofilm and therefore might be useful to control oral infectious microorganisms in dental plaque.

Nagayoshi et al.[11] in this year 2004 the effect of ozonated water against E. faecalis and S. mutans infections in dentin of freshly extracted bovine incisors After treating with ozonated water, the number of colony forming units (CFU) of bacteria in the infected dentin chips was significantly decreased fluorescence microscopic analysis showed an increase of membrane permeability of S. mutans cells, meaning that ozonated water had a strong bactericidal effect against bacteria invading dentinal tubules of root canals.

Hems et al.[12] in this year 2005 to evaluate the potential of ozone as an antibacterial agent using E. faecalis as the test species. The antibacterial efficacy of ozone was tested against both broth and biofilm cultures. Ozone was sparged for 30, 60, 120 and 240 s, through overnight broth cultures of E. faecalis and compared with those that were centrifuged, washed and resuspended in water in a separate test, biofilms were also exposed to gaseous ozone sodium hypochlorite (NaOCl) was used as a positive control. All experiments were repeated four times. They came to the conclusion that NaOCl was found to be superior to ozonated water in killing E. faecalis in broth culture and in biofilms.

Huth et al.[13] in this year 2006 to evaluate cytotoxicity of gaseous and aqueous ozone. Cytotoxicity of gaseous and aqueous ozone on human oral epithelial cells and gingival fibroblast cells compared with established antiseptics over a time of 1 min, and compared with the antibiotic, metronidazole, over 24. They came to the conclusion that Aqueous ozone revealed the highest level of biocompatibility of the tested antiseptic.

Estrela et al.[14] in this year 2006 to evaluate the antimicrobial potential of ozone applied to three different solutions in an ultrasonic cleaning system against Staphylococcus aureus. Solutions used in an ultrasonic cleaning system sterile distilled water Vinegar and sterile distilled water Endozime AWpluz. They came to the conclusion that Bacterial growth was not observed in any of the experimental solutions when ozone was added.

Polydorou et al.[15] in this year 2006 to evaluate the antibacterial effect of two different application times of ozone gas on an in vitro infected cavity model, the antimicrobial effect of both bonding systems and 80 s of ozone was significantly higher than the 40 s ozone. They came to the conclusion that Longer exposure to ozone has a strong bactericidal effect on microorganisms within the dentinal tubules of deep cavities, which could result in increasing the clinical success of restoration.

Celiberti et al[16] in this year 2006 to assess the effects of the highly reactive molecule of ozone on sound enamel physical properties and its effects on sealing ability. To assess the effects of the highly reactive molecule of ozone on sound enamel physical properties and its effects on sealing ability The effect of ozone gas (HealOzone, KaVo, 2100 ppm for 40 s) was evaluated prior to etching and sealing on sound enamel physical properties, including knoop surface microhardness, contact angle (free surface energy of enamel), acid resistance, and sealing ability. They came to the conclusion that ozone can be applied as a prophylactic treatment prior to etching and the placement of sealant.

Muller P et al.[17] in this year 2007 to assess the antimicrobial potential of ozone gas and photodynamic therapy (PDT) in vitro. Sixty-second application of gasiform vacuum-ozone or vacuum alone (on wet or air-dried biofilm samples, PDT (i.e., methylene blue in combination with or without a diode soft laser, and a soft laser alone), antimicrobial solutions: immersion of biofilms for 60 s in 0.2% and 2% chlorhexidine or in 0.5% and 5% hypochlorite solution. They came to the conclusion that gasiform ozone and PDT had a minimal effect on the viability of microorganisms organised in a cariogenic biofilm.

Kshitish & Laxman.[18] in this year 2010 to evaluate and to compare the effects of irrigating ozonated water (0.082 mg/h for 5-10 minutes) and 0.2% chlorhexidine (Control group) in clinical parameters such as gingival index and gingival bleeding index, in addition to the action of ozone on oral microorganisms. Author came in conclusion that reduction of the gingival index and bleeding index in the ozone group was significant in comparison to chlorhexidine. Ozone is a powerful agent in the inactivation of microorganisms associated to periodontitis.

Skurska et al.[19] in this year 2010 a comparison of the clinical condition and salivary levels of matrix metalloproteinase after scaling and root planning or ozone therapy in patients with aggressive or chronic periodontitis. They came in conclusion that the scaling and root planning combined with ozone therapy does not contribute to further improvement in clinical periodontal parameters in patients with aggressive and chronic periodontitis. Ozone therapy combined with SRP leads to a decrease of saliva matrix metalloproteinase concentration in patients with aggressive periodontitis.

Dhingra et al.[20] in this year 2011 to evaluate the clinical effects of a single subgingival irrigation with ozonated water on gingival inflammation in orthodontic patients and also to correlate the clinical effects with LDH enzyme activity in GCF. They came to the conclusion that at the end of one month, a single subgingival irrigation of 0.01 mg) ozonated water could effectively reduce the gingival inflammation in orthodontic patients. Thus, subgingival ozone irrigation can be an effective method that can be performed during monthly visits on orthodontic patients to reduce the gingival inflammation because of plaque-retentive orthodontic appliances.

El Hadary et al.[21] in this year 2011 to evaluate the effects of ozonated oil under the influence of Cyclosporine A in bone integration of dental implants. Group A: treated with ozonated oil (sunflower oil) 0.550 ml in gel applied to fill each osteotomy site for the implant. Group B: non-ozonated (Control group). They came to the conclusion that the administration of short-term cyclosporine together with the topical application of ozonated oil may influence bone density.

Huth et al.[22] in this year 2011 to investigate the antimicrobial effectiveness of aqueous and gaseous ozone in comparison to the antiseptic chlorhexidine digluconate on periodontal microorganisms in planktonic state and in biofilm. Aqueous ozone reduced 99% of the total A. actinomycetemcomitans in planktonic state and 70% in biofilm. Gaseous ozone(1-16gm-3) reduced Aggregatibacter actinomycetemcomitans (A.a) 99.7% in isolated state and 70% in biofilm (53 g m^3). They came in conclusion that gaseous ozone presented greater antimicrobial activity against aggregatibacter actinomycetemcomitans. Chlorhexidine, aqueous and gaseous ozone showed dose dependent effectiveness; however, there was greater efficacy in planktonic bacteria than in biofilm.

Hauser-Gerspach et al.[23] in this year 2012 to investigate the antimicrobial efficacy of gaseous ozone on bacteria adhered to several surfaces of titanium and zirconium, and also to evaluate the adhesion of osteoblast-like M G-63 cells to surfaces that were treated with ozone. They came to the conclusion that ozone did not affect the surface structures of the test specimens and did not influence osteoblastic cells proliferation negatively. Polished titanium and zirconium (acid etched and polished) presented lower bacterial colonization.

Kronenberg et al.[24] in this year 2012 evaluating whether there is no difference in the anticaries protection of ozone and cervitec/fluorine around the brackets, in addition to assess whether diagnodent and the quantity of induced fluorescent light are not superior to the visual evaluation of initial carious lesions. They came to conclusion that anticaries protective effect of Cervitec/Fluorine during the placement of the orthodontic appliance was superior to ozone.

Chandra et al.[25] in this year 2013 to evaluate the success of root filling with zinc oxide – ozonated oil and and zinc oxide eugenol in primary molar. Author concludes that ozonated oil- ZnO demonstrated a good clinical and radiographic success at 12th months follow up visits and it can be considered as an alternative obturating material in infected primary teeth.

Beretta et al.[26] in this year 2017 to assess the effectiveness of a new protocol for deep caries treatment in deciduous teeth based on: 1) the incomplete removal of carious dentin tissue; 2) the use of new technology (ozone) for the disinfection of carious dentine; 3) the creation of a peripheral seal in healthy tissue for bonding procedures with rubber dam isolation. They came to the conclusion that the use of ozone, proved to be an excellent alternative, with the fundamental advantage of saving dental tissue and preventing the invasion of the pulp chamber.

Kucuk et al.[27] in this year 2021 to assess the cytotoxicity of various concentrations of ozonated water (OW) on human primary dental pulp cells s, cells were divided into 6 experimental groups; four groups of OW in concentrations of 2 mg/L, 4 mg/L, 8 mg/L, and 16 mg/L, untreated control group, and cell culture without cells. Cytotoxicity was evaluated after exposure for 5-min exposure using Mosmann's Tetrazolium Toxicity (MTT) assay at 0 h and 48 h time points it could be concluded that the ozonated water is non-toxic and induces proliferation of cells as well. Tis proliferation effect was time and dose-dependent.

Luppieri et al.[28] in this year 2022 to evaluate the effectiveness of ozone therapy in (1) increasing the compactness of decayed dentin (main aim), (2) reducing dentin hypersensitivity, (3) decreasing the salivary bacterial count, and (4) improving the quality of life in ECC-affected children during a 3-month follow-up They came to the conclusion that ozone therapy may be considered an effective technique for treating ECC-affected teeth in preschool children uncooperative with traditional restorative treatments since it helps to slow down the caries progression and improve patients' quality of life. Moreover, being a simple and non-invasive technique, it may help children to become used to dental treatments.

Hamid et al.[29] in this year 2023 to evaluate the histological Assessment of the Oral Soft Tissue Regenerative Capacity of Hyaluronic Acid and Ozonated Oil. They came to the conclusion that topical use of PerioKIN Hyaluronic 1% gel and O3OHEAL-M gel three times daily for secondary intention wounds give a satisfying result of healing and isolation to get rid of the infection and ugly scar in appropriate time, so we recommend using it as an auxiliary medication for tissue loss wounds.

Discussion

Indications

- **Dental Caries:** The gaseous or aqueous form of ozone eliminates the acidogenic bacteria by decarboxylation of pyruvic acid which is produced by acidogenic bacteria to acetic acid. The acetic acid causes the remineralization of carious lesion and also buffers plaque due to high Pka values.[30]
- **Restoration:** The protocol proposed starts with dental isolations using a rubber dam, then layer of carious dentin is removed. Ozone gas is then applied on the infected dentin that remains in the cavity for 60 sec with a single patient silicone cup. The longer exposure to ozone gas has a strong bactericidal effect on microorganisms with in the dentinal tubules of deep cavities. The objective of this procedure is to kill bacteria involved in the carious process like S – mutants and L – acidophilus.[31]
- **Hypersensitivity:** Ozone removes the smear layer, open up the dentinal tubules, broadens their diameter and allows the calcium and fluoride ions to flow into the dentinal tubules. easily, deeply and effectively to plug the dentinal tubules preventing the fluid exchange through these tubules.[30]
- **Gingivitis:** Fill the scaler fluid bottle with ozonated water (if applicable) and proceed with the scaling procedure. Apply ozonated oil and if needed slightly inside the sulcus at 400-600 IP with a sulcabrush. Provide the patient with ozonated oil for home use. Apply once or twice daily for few days.[12]
- **Periodontitis:** Highly significant improvement regarding pocket depth, plaque index, gingival index and bacterial count. Ozone is effective against many putative periodontopathogenic microorganism.[32]

- **Ozone therapy in tooth extraction:** Beneficial effect in the treatment of the refractory osteomyelitis, as adjunct with antibiotics surgery and hyperbaric oxygen. used in management of bone necrosis and extraction sites during and after oral surgery by stimulating cell proliferation and soft tissue healing.[33]

  Ozone therapy in tooth extraction- Proceed with tooth removal. Flush the socket with ozonated water. Cover the site with a gauze, use an applicator tip to irrigate with ozone gas (40-80 μg/NmL, 1-2 min) while suctioning excess gas. Fill the socket with few drops of ozonated oil. Home use ozonated oil once or twice daily and decrease application according to the healing phase.[33]

- **Effect of ozone therapy in wound healing:** Ozone accelerates the healing of soft tissue conditions like apthous ulcers, herpes labialis ANUG and other gum infections. Ozone causes the synthesis of biologically active substance like interleukins, leukotrienes and prostaglandin which is beneficial in reducing inflammation and wound healing. Most mild soft tissue lesions, ulcers and wounds respond favorably with home use of ozonated water and oil (PI 600-800). In severe cases, in-office ozone gas/water application.[34]

- **Peri- implantitis:** Powerful antimicrobial agent that kills the microorganism causing periimplantitis. A positive wound healing effect due to increase in tissue circulation. Sterile the surface of both the implant and bone. Initiate the reparative mechanism allowing tissue regeneration around implant surface.[35]
- **Ozone therapy in oral prophylaxis:** Fill the scaler fluid bottle with ozonated water (if applicable) and proceed with the scaling procedure. Irrigate at demand with ozonated water. Ozonated oils if needed.[34]

- **Dental unit water system:** Dental Unit Water Lines **DUWL-** is becoming a major concern for at-risk patients and dental staff exposed to contaminated dental unit water and aerosols via ingestion or inhalation, as well as potential infection of surgical wounds. Infection control agencies recommend that DUWL should not exceed the maximum allowable colony-forming-units (CFU) of drinking water, ranging from 100 to 500 CFU/mL. Reports of heavily biofilm -contaminated DUWL where a cohort of microorganisms (heterotrophic bacteria, fungi, amoebae, protozoa, coliforms, Legionella, pseudomonas viruses) were found and the total bacterial count was at hundreds of thousand CFUs. Ozone achieved a 57% reduction in biofilm and 65% reduction in viable bacteria inspite of being used in very low doses and with a short time of applications.[36]

- **Tooth brush contamination:** Most powerful antioxidant. Ozone application was found to remove toothbrush bristles microbiota following conventional brushing.[33]

Contraindications

1. Alcohol intoxication[37]
2. Ozone allergy[37]
3. Pregnancy [38]
4. Glucose -6 – phosphate dehydrogenase deficiency [39]
5. Hyperthyroidism-[40]

Do not drink alcohol directly before or after a session-At least wait 8 hours after your last drink before going for an ozone therapy session, and at least 4 hours after the session before having a drink again. Ozone and heat will increase blood circulation and alcohol thins out blood which can lead to additional strain on your heart.[37]

Pregnancy. Ozone therapy has been used with good results in the treatment of different diseases associated with pregnancy such as: placental insufficiency, fetal growth retardation, cervical ectopy, preeclampsia. However, it should be avoided during the first trimester of pregnancy (0-13 weeks), a critical time for development of the embryo and fetus.[38]

Glucose-6-phosphate-dehydrogenase deficiency (G-6-PD) (favism): The enzyme G-6-PD is crucial for eliminating equivalents able to abolish excessive oxidation and intensive hemolysis. Deficiency of the same, results in hemolytic disease known as favism. On exposure to ozone, it is associated with the precipitation of acute hemolysis in such cases.[39]

Hyperthyroidism: The sensitivity of the lung to damage due to ozone therapy may be highly dependent on an individual's thyroid hormone status. The chances of aggravation of the lung toxicity in patients with a hyperthyroid state are more likely.[40]

Various form and routes of ozone administration

- Ozone is dispensed in various forms such as ozonated water, ozonated gas or ozonated oil. These forms are used either in combination or singly for the dental treatments.

There are different ozone generating systems:[41]

- UV system
- Cold plasma system
- Corona discharge system

UV system:[42]

- This system emits UV light at 185 nm
- Produce low ozone concentrations.
- The oxygen molecule absorbs light energy when exposed to ultraviolet light and dissociated. Later, the oxygen atoms react with other oxygen molecules to form ozone.
- Used in aesthetics, air and water purifications.

Corona discharge system:[42]

- Produce high concentration of ozone by directly using power dissipation.
- Ozone is formed by electrical discharge which is convert into ozone.
- It is a most common used in the medical /dental field.
- It is easy to handle and it has a controlled ozone production rate.

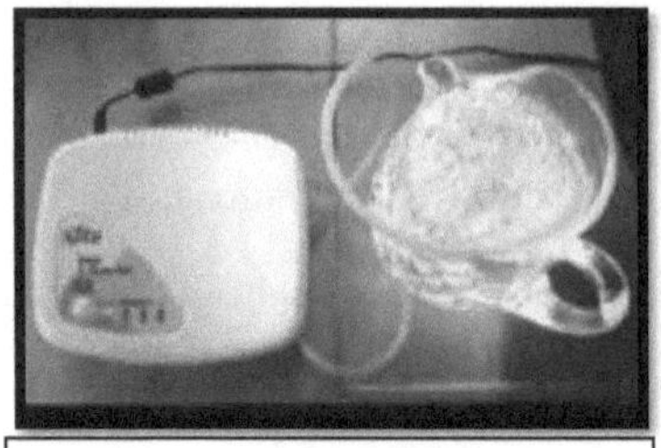

Figure-1 A Medical Grade Oxygen Fed Corona Discharge Ozone Unit[43]

Cold plasma system[42]

- In this system am electrostatics field is created between the anode and the cathode rods.
- It is used in air and water purification.

Product	System used	Form	Advantages	Disadvantages
Ozonette DENT (Sold by Sedecal)[11]	Corona discharge system	Gaseous form	1. Handheld syringe application. 2. Ozone flow rate and concentration can be adjusted with uniform distribution. 3. AOD 4. Ozone is removed by the double independent circuit with two internal catalysts. 5. Compatible with O2 cylinder.	1. Uneconomical.
Ozonytron-XPO (MIO Int. OZONYTRON GmbH)[12]	Cold plasma system	Gaseous form	1. Application through – Plasma electrode/nozzle/mouth tray 2. Can be used in various treatment modalities (disinfection of cavities, root canals, gingival pockets) along with in office/internal bleaching with different applicators provided. 3. Mouth Tray, encloses the targeted area from the oral cavity, preventing inhalation of ozone plasma.	1. Chances of leakage with plasma electrode; thus be used with saliva ejector. 2. Plasma is directly generated at the treatment site, creating microcurrent. Thus contraindicated in • Epileptic patient • Cardiac pacemaker • Hypersensitivity to electric impulses.
Ozonsan cytozon (Hansler Medical)[13]	Normobaric infusion therapy (ozonized water)	Aqueous form	1. Application through handpick or water outlet tap. 2. Additional bayonet connection allows multiple connections of devices such as ultrasonic devices or piezosurgery 3. Ease of handling 4. Safe handling 5. Painless treatment modality.	1. Less effective when compared to gaseous ozone.
OxActiv (ozonated olive oil gel)[14]	Infused ozone in gel based product	Aqueous gel	1. Ease of application 2. Safe handling 3. Cost-effective 4. Ease of availability.	1. Least effective when compared to all the other modalities discussed above.

Figure – 2 AOD: Automatic overpressure detection. Manufacture of ozone in dentistry [44]

Routes of Ozone Administrations

- Ozonated oil– ozonated oils are naturally derivatives of plant extracts. Mycobacterium, Staphylococci, Streptococci, Enterococci, Pseudomonas and Escherichia coli are all susceptible to ozonated oil (Oleozone and Bioperoxile).[45]

Ozonated water – ozonated aqueous form can be used as:[46]

- Disinfectant
- Sterilizing agent
- Irrigation solution
- Haemostatic agent

Ozonated gas or gaseous form- Gaseous ozone can be administered topically by an open or sealed suction system to avoid inhalation and possible adverse effects.[47]

It is most frequently used method.[47]

It is conservative and non – invasive therapy which is used in the treatment of dental caries and hypomineralized teeth.[47]

Healozone by KaVo-employs an air-based system wherein gas is used in a closed circuit. The concentration of ozone delivered to tissue is 2100ppm. Good air tightness of the cap is required for the ozone application.[48]

OzonyTron by MYMED – A glass camera forms the glass probe comprised of noble gases which conduct and emit electromagnetic energy. High frequency and voltage are used in this appliance. Energy is emitted on the tissue with an ozone concentration of 10-100ug/ml. Hence, can also be applied to unreacheable area of oral cavity.[49]

Product photo (Prozone) by Wand H-

- Prozone customized dosage according to the use in oral surgery and restoration. It provides a clean and hygienic procedure because of the disposable plastic attachments.[49]

Ozotop-

- It is small unit, utilizing a corona discharge mechanism and provides a free gas flow. This is an open system and required high volume suction during the procedure[49].
- It can easily penetrate the periodontal pocket and root canal system[49].
- Ozone is applied for 6,12,18 and 24 sec depending on the use[49].
- Surgical disinfectant takes 12 sec and periodontal disinfectant takes 18sec[49].

Mechanism of Action of Ozone

Antimicrobial effects-

Ozone helps in killing of both types of gram-positive bacteria and gram-negative bacteria such as Pseudomonas aeruginosa and E – coli (According to microbiology research data).[50]

The antimicrobial effect of ozone produces by the action on cell by damaging its cytoplasmic membrane due to ozonolysis of dual bond.[50]

Acc to thanomsub et al. they demonstrated the effect of ozone treatment on cell growth and structural changes in bacteria including E-coli salmonella species, staphylococcus aureus and bacillus. Ozone is very efficient in antibiotics resistant strains. And its antimicrobial activity increase in liquid environment especially in acidic PH.[50]

Immunostimulating Action-

Ozone influences cellular and humoral immune system. It stimulates proliferation of immunocompetent cells and phagocytosis. It also activates function of macrophages and increases sensitivity of microorganism to phagocytosis. The production of interleukin-2 launches an entire cascade of subsequent immunological reaction that's means ozone is very useful for immune activation in patient with low immune deficit or immune status.[51]

Anti – inflammatory and analgesic action-

Ozone therapy help in reducing pain, inflammation and discomfort by the action of Leukotrienes, prostaglandins and interleukin.[52]

It enhances local blood microcirculation, oxygen delivery to the tissues and it eliminate toxin.[52] Ozone is negative charge (basic) and infection or inflammation is positive charge (acidic) so the chemistry of infection and inflammation attracts ozone to the area.[52]

Anti-hypoxic action-

Ozone has been shown to elevate the pO2 levels in tissues and improve oxygen transportation throughout. In repetitive low doses, it protects the calls against oxygen free radicals by activating various enzymes such as superoxide dismutases, catalases, dehydrogenases, and glutathione. It also prevents the aggravation of erythrocytes and increases the contact surface area for the attachment of oxygen, for better transportation. Ozone also improves the metabolism of inflamed tissues by reducing local inflammation and potentiating the oxidation process.[53]

Biosynthetic action-

By influencing the biochemical processes within the cells, it stimulates protein synthesis and thus increases the amounts of ribosomes and mitochondria within. At the cellular level, this explains the regenerative potentiality of the tissues and organs post-ozone therapy. It also aids in the activation of angiogenesis.[54]

Safety – Precautions

- The use of ozone gas intra-orally is probably the most critical among all other ozone applications in industry and healthcare when it comes to inadvertent and accidental inhalation of ozone gas. Thus, it is paramount for the dentist and his/her staff to take all necessary safety precautions during the application of ozone gas intra-orally to avoid any accidental inhalation.[55]
- Stop immediately the procedure if the particular odor of ozone is detected. Check for leaks and application modality.[55]
- Whenever possible, use a silicone cup (i.e. a piece of 10, 8, 6 mm ø silicone tube adapted to the delivery handpiece) when applying ozone gas.[55]
- At all times, use the dental unit high vacuum to suction any gas leaking outside the silicone cup or the treatment area even if the delivery handpiece has a dedicated suction pump.[55]
- Be certain that vitamin C in single gram increments and medical grade oxygen with a concentrator mask are always available in the dental office. In case of an accidental inhalation of ozone gas, mild to severe coughing may occur. If possible, have the patient consume the vitamin C in a cup of water. Next, have the patient breath the oxygen delivered at flow rate of 2 L/min. If coughing is still evident after 15 min, administer another gram of vitamin C. If two rounds of vitamin C administration fail to resolve the coughing or if oral administration is not possible, a doctor should be prepared to administer via sublingual, a misting inhaler, intramuscular or intravenous routes; however intravenous and intramuscular administration should not be attempted by an inexperienced doctor.[55]

Ozone Therapy in Caries Management

- Dental caries is defined as a chronic infectious disease with multifactorial etiology. The putative pathogen of dental caries is S. mutans. Preventive measures aiming to control active and inactive caries progression are focused on developing strategies to reduce a load of this microorganism in the oral biofilm.[56]

  The S. mutans cariogenic potential resides in four core attributes.[57]

  (i) Adherence to enamel surface.

  (ii) Production of acidic metabolites.

  (iii) The capacity to build up glycogen reserves.

  (iv) The capacity to synthesize extracellular polysaccharides.

S. mutant behaviors with ozonated water (Extracted carious tooth)

- The in vitro antimicrobial activity procedure was performed by using ozonated water. Commercial oral water jet (Aqualab, Sweden Martina, Milan, Italy); was used as an ozonated water generator device following the manufacturer's instructions. This system was able to produce different ozonated water formulations, respectively: 0.025; 0.042; 0.060 [O3] mg/L.[58]
- The experiment was performed in triplicate by using different Eppendorf tubes, each tube contained 100µL of S. mutans inoculum in Schaedler broth. Then, immediately 2mL of ozonated water containing the different ozone concentrations added. After vigorous mixing, each formulation was inoculated on the surface of a petri dish containing 15mL of Schaedler agar. The colonies formed after 48h of incubation at 37°C with 5% CO2 were counted.[58]

The results shown in Figure reveal an effective and synergic activity by using the maximum O3 concentration [0.06mg/L] plus light in a wavelength range from 450 to 470 nm. This experiment also showed that the photodynamic treatment is

ineffective if we use O3 at a lower concentrations range [0.042mg/L], in fact, in these conditions, the biofilm inhibition is comparable with only ozone use.[58]

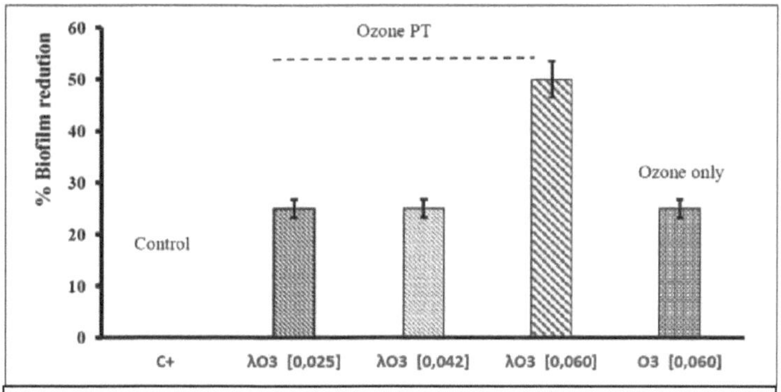

Figure -3 Different ozone concentrations[58]

Percentage of S. mutans mature biofilm reduction evaluated with different ozone concentrations and light in a wavelength range from 450 to 470 nm.

Ozone Therapy in Cavity Disinfectant

Removing infected dentine is a routine protocol for the treatment of dental caries but there is no certain way to be sure if there are bacterial remains on the cavity surface or not. Even if affected dentine has removed, bacterial component may have still existed by the depth of 0.1-2.4 mm from cavity floor, through the pulp tissue.[59-60]

To prevent pulp tissue from bacterial invasion which may still exist in cavity after treatment or comes from microleakage between restorative filling materials and dentine tissue; cavity cleansing systems have been considered to be used in dental practice for a long time ago.[61-62]

Ozone treatment that has been using in dentistry due to its antibacterial activity, new tissue forming capacity and the ability of stimulating healing. Ozone gas is the most effective anti-oxidant agent in nature.[63]

Ozonized water and ozone gas reduce the total cultivable microbiota significantly in vitro.Baysan et al. found a significant reduction in S. mutans and Streptecoccus sobrinus in the ozone-treated side of the root caries lesions.[65] Application of ozone (OzonyTronX) has also been proposed due to its antibacterial activity.[64]

Procedure-

All teeth surfaces except caviteted areas were cleaned with savlon solutions and washed with saline solution. After that, superficial surfaces of necrotic dentin were removed with sterile steel round burs.[65]

Cavities were prepared by a depth of 2,5 mm to make enough place for compomer restorative materials. Remained dentin was cleaned with ozonated water solution and dried with cotton pellets. For microbiological assessment, dentine samples were collected with cooled burs from the middle of cavity floor.[65]

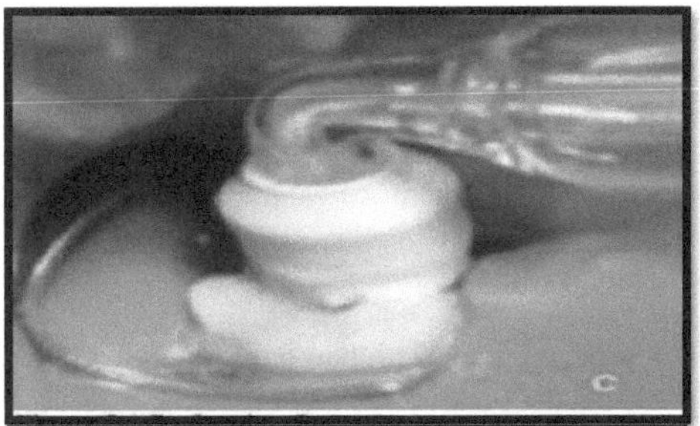

Figure -4 OzonyTronX was applied for 3 seconds in forth degree with CA Prob.[65]

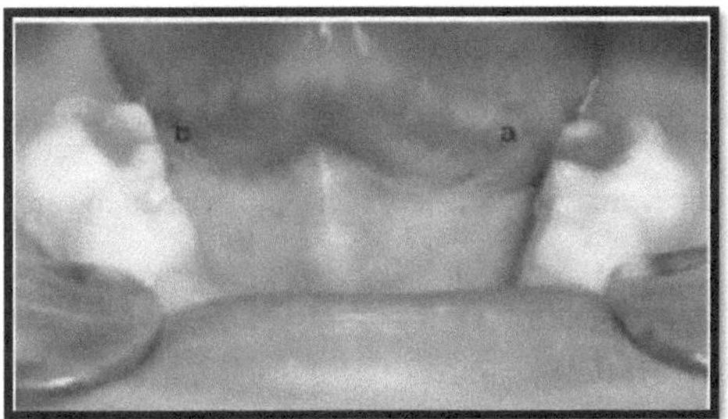

Figure – 5 Ozonated water in cavities[65]

Ozony TronX

After a period of four weeks, compomer restorations were removed from the cavities by means of a sterile diamond bur without contacting the dentine on cavity walls. Then, the dentine samples were collected for a second time by sterile steel round burs. A total CFU count was obtained through a culture (MSA plates) of dentine sample collect. **Author conclude thar total CFU count decrease after ozone therapy application**.[65]

Ozone Therapy for Deep Dental Caries Treatment

The **American Academy of Pediatric Dentistry** has established that "the objectives of restorative treatment are to repair or limit damage from caries, protect and preserve tooth structure, re-establish adequate function, restore aesthetics (where applicable).[66]

A new protocol for deep caries treatment in deciduous teeth based on: The incomplete removal of carious dentin tissue; 2) the use of new technology (ozone) for the disinfection of carious dentine; 3) the creation of a peripheral seal in healthy tissue for bonding procedures with rubber dam isolation.[66]

In recent years the use of new technologies for the treatment of tooth decay in young patients has revolutionized the world of pediatric dentistry. New approaches to ultra-conservative treatment of deciduous teeth include the use of ozone gas.[67]

The studies were resumed in the 80s, when Dr. Edward Lynch of the Royal London Hospital Medical College demonstrated how a carious lesion exposed to a single application of the gas could re-mineralized [Lynch, 2004].[68]

Later in recent years, the introduction of new devices has made it possible to apply gas directly on the tooth surfaces affected by early caries, special single-patient silicon cups [Baysan and Lynch, 2006]. The first device for dental use, after obtaining a vacuum inside the silicon cup mounted on the dedicated handpiece, was capable of delivering pure ozone starting from ambient air.[69]

Recently a new device (Healozone X4*) was developed which is able to produce ozone taking it from a special canister of O2, and transform it into a concentration of 32 g/m3, with efficacy and power much higher than earlier devices.[66]

The use of ozone has often focused on decontamination of carious dentin, especially in deciduous teeth of very small or non-cooperative patients, followed by the application of various products in order to obtain the re-mineralization of the surfaces [Samuel et al., 2016].[70]

Procedure:

The protocol consists of the following:[66]

- Partial removal of carious dentin.
- Sterilization of the remaining tissue by ozone.
- Composite restoration under isolation of the operative field with a rubber dam.

The operating sequence applied in all restorations was the following

Isolation of the working area with rubber dam (limited to teeth E-D with hook on the most distal tooth). Removal of the top layer of carious dentin using rosette burs, without uncovering the pulp tissue. Ozone application on the infected dentin for 60 s with single-patient silicone cup (Healozone™ X4). Vestibular and lingual walls with this material were created to allow the correct positioning of the silicone cup, because Healozone is not able to to deliver gas without a complete vacuum inside the cup, which must be obtained by an adequate seal of the cup itself.[66] 3-step technique bonding (etching, primer, bonding), restoration of the decayed tooth with composite resins and polishing and occlusion check.[66]

The presence of the following 6 items defined success.[66]

- Restoration still in place.
- Absence of marginal microleakage.
- Absence of the restoration fractures.
- Presence of an interproximal contact (for Class II cavities).
- Absence of discoloration.
- Absence of pain.

Ozone Therapy in Dentin Hypersensitivity

Dentin hypersensitivity (DH) is characterized as an acute and brief pain when dentin is exposed to thermal, evaporative, tactile, osmotic, or chemical stimuli and cannot be attributed to any form of dental defect or pathology (Canadian Advisory Board on Dentin Hypersensitivity, 2003; Cunha-Cruz, et al., 2011). It is a pain that disappears immediately after the removal of the generating stimulus (Sobral & Garone, 1999).[71]

The most accepted theory to explain cervical dentinal hypersensitivity is the "hydrodynamic theory", in which the rapid movement of fluid inside the dentinal tubules stimulates odontoblasts and nerve cells present inside the tubules or even in the pulp chamber. Thus, with the increase of hydrodynamic stimuli inside the tubules, the nociceptives are activated, causing the characteristic pain (Brännström & Garberoglia 1980, Moretzsohn & Campos, 2001).[72-73]

According to (Mastrantonio & Ramalho in this year 2003) the decrease in dentin hypersensitivity level after treatment by both oils may be due to the presence of polyurethane in their compositions.[74]

According to (Goldberg, et al., 2011; Zhang, et al., 2019**.** It has been shown that polyurethane can induce bone neoformation in addition to the formation of collagen and mineralized tissue (matrix of collagen and hydroxyapatite crystals) which makes it biocompatible with dentin, which also has hydroxyapatite crystals and fibers in its collagen composition.[75]

According to (Veena, et al., 2020) in this in vitro study observed that adjuvant application of a desensitizing agent containing arginine, with ozonized oil, had a synergistic effect, where the latter causes the opening of the dentinal tubules allowing a more compact penetration of the former and, therefore, can be an approach of potentially more effective treatment in the management of dentin hypersensitivity.[76]

Procedure:

- Patients with complaints of dentin hypersensitivity in daily activities dentin hypersensitivity were selected.[77]
- Ozonated oil were applied on sensitive area of teeth in the quantity of 0.5ml only once for 5 minutes with the aid of a micro brush and under relative isolation with cotton wool rolls. Then, the tooth was dried with gauze.[77]
- **Dentin hypersensitivity was stimulated** through evaporative and thermal tests. The thermal test was done by applying cold flexible cotton swabs at cervical area of the teeth for 3 seconds. The air jet was applied to each tooth for 3 seconds at 0.5 cm distance, with neighboring teeth isolated with utility wax.[77]
- All the results were recorded in the individual patient record.[77]

Evaluation parameter –

- Dentin hypersensitivity level was measured using a numerical rating scale, ranging from 0 to 10. After each stimulus, the evaluator asked which number on the scale best represented the pain the patient felt at the time of the tests.[77]
- **Authors concluded that ozonated oil was effective for the treatment of dentin hypersensitivity.**[77]

Management of Gingival Inflammation in Orthodontics Patients with Ozonated Water Irrigation

Adequate levels of plaque control are difficult to achieve in patients with fixed orthodontic appliances. As a result, orthodontic patients often develop gingivitis, with the response characterized by gingival inflammation and hyperplasia.[78]

Lactate dehydrogenase is an enzyme that is normally limited to the cytoplasm of cells, and it is only released extracellularly after cell death. Lactate dehydrogenase (LDH) in gingival crevicular fluid (GCF) is significantly correlated with gingival inflammation (17–19) and tissue destruction.[79-80]

Treatment Procedure:

The orthodontics patients were subjected to full-mouth irrigation with ozonated water (along with the use of suction device) that was released from an irrigation device, 'Kent ozone Dental Jet TY-820'. The device released a single pulsating stream of ozonated water from the nozzle that could be adjusted for different speeds and pressures ranging from 66 to 130 kPa (kilo pascals) and an ozone output of 0.1 mg l)1 (0.1 ppm), at a noise output of <70 dB (decibels) and water outflow of 280–420 ml.

To facilitate subgingival ozone irrigation, a 20-gauge blunt needle was bent and attached to the tip of the nozzle of the ozone dental jet holder. A stop clock was used to set the irrigation time to 15 s at each site, after which the irrigation was stopped total time of 5–10 min was spent for irrigation for each patient.[20]

After irrigation, the patients were instructed to perform regular oral hygiene habits, twice daily brushing for a minimum of 2 min, using a standard tooth brush (Colgate Super Flexible with medium consistency bristles) and tooth paste (Colgate dental cream) provided to them. The patients were dispersed and instructed to report on the subsequent 14th day. The procedure of assessment of clinical indices and PPD was then repeated on the 14th and 28th day.[20]

At the end of one month, a single subgingival irrigation of 0.01 mg l) ozonated water could effectively reduce the gingival inflammation in orthodontic patients. Thus, subgingival ozone irrigation can be an effective method that can be performed during monthly visits on orthodontic patients to reduce the gingival inflammation because of plaque-retentive orthodontic appliances.[20]

Ozone Therapy in Management of Chronic Periodontitis

Periodontitis is a multi -factorial disease of which bacterial plaque is recognized as the main etiologic agent in the initiation and progression of periodontitis.[81]

Ozone has been recently advocated as an irrigating agent predominantly due to its antimicrobial action which results from oxidation of microbial cellular components and altering the sub gingival homeostasis. The antimicrobial action is by direct reactions of molecular ozone and other a free radical mediated reaction.[82]

Procedure

Irrigation Protocol -

The periodontitis sites were subjected to ozonized water subgingival irrigation. The subgingival irrigation device (Kent Ozone Dental Jet TY 820 Kent Ro Systems Ltd, Noida, India) fitted with a modified subgingival tip was inserted 3mm deep into the pocket. The pocket was irrigated for one minute.[82]

The device released a single pulsating stream of ozonized water from the nozzle with a water outflow of ≥150ml/min with ozone output of 0.082 mg/h. Microbiologic sampling were repeated at the test sites.[82]

The patients were recalled at the first, second and third weeks. After 4 weeks patients were reviewed and clinical parameters were recorded and microbiologic sampling was done at the test and control sites.[82]

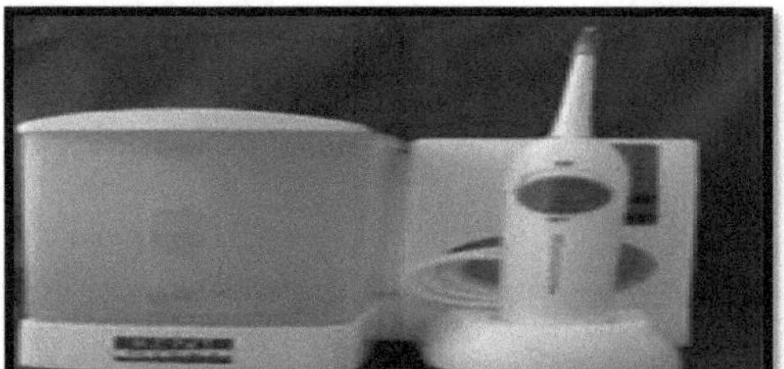

Figure -6 Kent Ozone Dental Jet[82]

Collection of subgingival plaque sample and microbiological analysis

After removing supra gingival plaque, tooth was isolated with sterile cotton rolls. Three sterile fine endodontic paper points (No. 40) were inserted to the depth of each study periodontal pocket for 30 seconds, and transferred to 10 ml of thioglycollate media.[82] Microbiologic samples were vortxed in a vortex mixer and subsequently incubated for two hours. The samples were then serially diluted. 100μl of the diluted specimen was spread with a sterile L shaped spreader onto brain heart infusion agar and anerobically cultured using anerobic jar (MERK) with anerobic generator Anacult A (Gas Pack) at 35-37°C for 5 days. All the samples were then inspected for total anerobic colony count, using the digital colony counter.[82]

Ozonized water subgingival irrigation can improve the clinical and microbiological parameters in patients with chronic periodontitis when used as an adjunct to scaling and root planning.[82]

Ozone Therapy in Dental Surgery

In dental surgery, ozone may be useful to promote hemostasis, enhance the local oxygen supply, and inhibit bacterial growth.[85] Ozone can react with blood components (erythrocytes, leukocytes, platelets, endothelial cells, and the vascular system) and positively affect oxygen metabolism, cell energy, the immunomodulatory effect, antioxidant defense system, and microcirculation in the tissue.[84-85]

Methods:

All patients were instructed to avoid any anti-inflammatory drugs or antibiotics 12 h prior to the procedure.[86]

Extractions were carried out under local anesthesia via the buccal guttering technique after adequate elevation and reflection of a buccal mucoperiosteal flap. Ozone therapy was performed using an ozone generator (Ozonytron; Biozonix GmbH, Germany) with a high frequency 7.5 cm deep tissue probe (Omega probe). The ozone generator was applied extra-orally at the insertion point of the masseter muscle immediately after surgery and on postoperative days 1, 3, 5, and 7, at an intensity of 80% for 10Ys.[86]

Evaluation

Pain was assessed on postoperative days 1, 3, 5, and 7 using a visual analogue scale (VAS) of 10 units in combination with a graphic rating scale. On the VAS, the leftmost end represented the absence of pain (score 0) and the rightmost end indicated the most severe pain (score 10).[86]

The degree of pain that the patients experienced on the study side (ozone application side) was significantly lower. Ozone application showed no benefits with regard to postoperative swelling.[86]

Effect of Ozone Therapy in Primary Tooth Obturation

Primary teeth with pulpal and periapical infections should be retained untile exfoliation whenever possible (Trairvorakul et al, 2008).[87]

The success of endodontics therapy in primary teeth depends mainly on the reduction or elimination of the bacteria from root canals by obturating materials having good antibacterial activity.[88]

The most commonly used root filling material are zinc oxide eugenol but he "wet" interface between ZOE paste and peri-radicular tissue allows the release of large quantities of eugenol into the apical tissue during a short time interval. At this higher concentration, eugenol has been proven to exhibit its cytotoxic effects.[89]

To overcome some of disadvantages. Ozone has been considered favorable, because it has some remarkable biological characteristics such as bactericidal action, debriding effect, angiogenesis stimulation capacity, and high oxidizing power.[9o]

Ozone could replace the eugenol content of ZOE with some other less irritating and biocompatible materials, an ideal obturating material. Obturating the root canal with a material with efficient antimicrobial efficacy as well as less toxicity might lead to an increase in treatment success.[91]

Procedure:

Primary molar with signs and symptoms indicating pulpectomy is required, which included.[28]

(a) Spontaneous pain or tenderness to percussion.

(b) Deep carious with pulp exposure.

(c) Uncontrolled hemorrhage after removal of coronal pulp tissue.

(d) Presence of a chronic apical abscess or sinus tract.

The radiographic characteristics included.[28]

(a) Coronal-radiographic evidence of a deep carious lesion or lesion approximating pulp.

(b) Discontinuity of lamina dura.

Under strict aseptic precautions, pulpectomy procedures were performed by a single operator. The teeth were anesthetized using lignocaine 2% with 1:80,000 epinephrine and isolated using a rubber dam. A proper access cavity was prepared using a straight fissure bur. The pulp was initially removed with spoon excavator, and further radicular pulp was removed with fine H-file along with repeated irrigation with chlorhexidine solution and saline. The root length was determined using a diagnostic radiograph.[28] The biomechanical preparation was done using K-files in a pull-back motion. Final irrigation was done using 1% sodium hypochlorite and normal saline. Each canal was enlarged to two or three instrument sizes greater than the first file used. The root canals were dried with cotton pellets and paper points and were ready for obturation.[28]Zinc oxide powder and ozonated sesame oil with a powder–liquid proportion of 4:1 mixed on a cool glass slab with the help of a stainless- steel spatula. The root canals were obturated using zinc oxide ozonated oil with the help of a Lentulo spiral.

Patient was recalled after 1 month and the final restoration was done with stainless steel crowns using standard techniques. After treatment, clinical evaluations were performed at 1, 6, and 12 months and radiographic evaluations were performed at 6 and 12 months.[28]**Ozonated oil-Zn-O demonstrated a good clinical and radiographic success at 12 months follow up visit and it can be considered as an alternative obturating material in infected primary teeth.[28]**

Effects of Ozone Therapy in Peri- Implantitis

Peri-implant diseases are described as inflammatory processes in the tissues surrounding implants in response to predominantly microbial biofilms on the surface of the implants.[92]

Peri-implant mucositis is defined as an inflammatory reaction triggered by microbial biofilms based on the parameter of bleeding on probing (BOP), without any loss of peri-implant bone, whereas peri-implantitis is characterized by BOP and/or suppuration with further loss of peri - implant bone.[93]

Since microbial biofilms play a major role in the etiology of peri-implant diseases, it has been considered that the elimination of microbial pathogens is mandatory for their treatment.[94]The objective of peri-implantitis therapy is to achieve inflammation resolution by decontaminating the implant surface, while preserving the implant-supporting tissues.[95]

Mckenna et al showed that gaseous ozone with or without hydrogen peroxide reduced plaque and bleeding scores around the soft tissues in patients with peri-implant mucositis. Their study also reported that the antimicrobial effect of ozone therapy could delay the advancement of peri-implant diseases.[96]

Implant surface decontamination procedures with ozone therapy:

At the peri-implantitis sites, mechanical debridement was performed using titanium curette. Ozone was applied to the peri-implantitis sites following mechanical debridement. The ozone delivery system was used the Ozone DTA Ozone Generator (DentaTec Dental AS, Hov, Norway). According to the manufacturer's information, OzoneDTA produces ozone at a fixed concentration of 2,100 ppm through a connected hand-piece.[97]

Ozone was delivered at 6 points circumferentially (2 mesial, 1 midbuccal, 1 midlingual, and 2 distal), for 30 seconds each, using a sterile, specially formed perio-tip. The perio-tip was halted 1 mm short of the pocket depth and ozone was applied as 80% oxygen for 30 seconds per day, 3 days a week, for 1 week. The implant surface decontamination procedures were repeated 3 times, on the starting date of the treatment (day 0), and then 2 days and 4 days later.[97]

The PBDs were filled with a bone substitute mixed with small pieces of CGF other 3 pieces of CGF were used as barrier membranes that were placed over the bone substitute. Non-resorbable sutures were used for the flap.[97]

Implant surface decontamination with the additional use of ozone therapy in SRT of peri-implantitis showed clinically and radiographically significant.[97]

Preoperative and postoperative clinical and radiographic views of the ozone group.

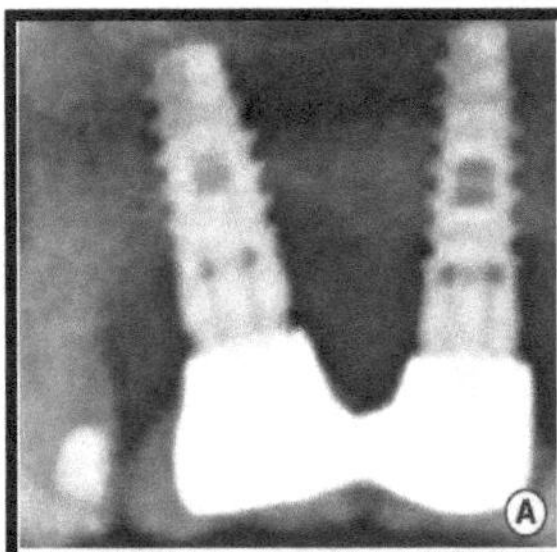

Figure-7 Radiographic view of the peri-implant bone defect at baseline.[97]

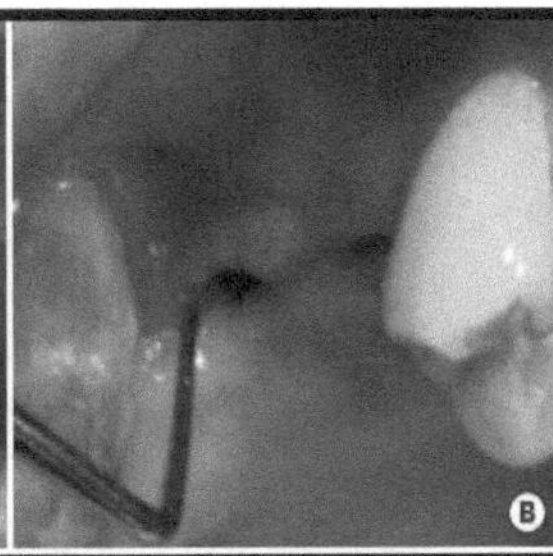

Figure -8 Probing of peri implantitis site baseline.[97]

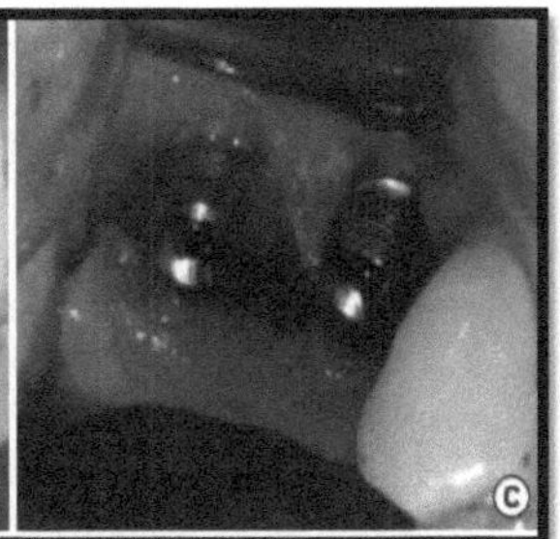

Figure- 9 Clinical defect configuration after flap elevation[97]

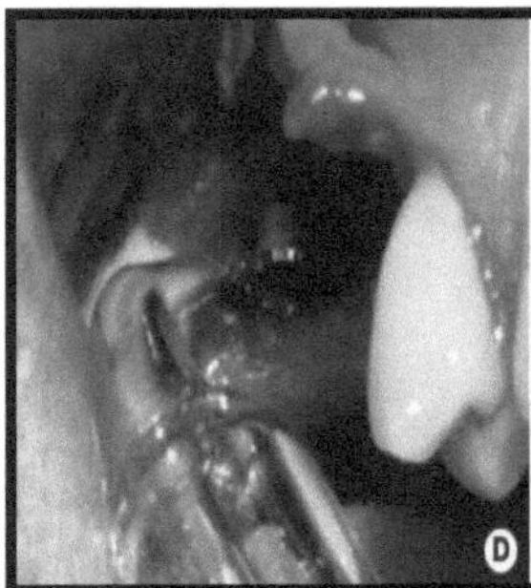

Figure – 10 Implant surface de - contamination using ozone therapy.[97]

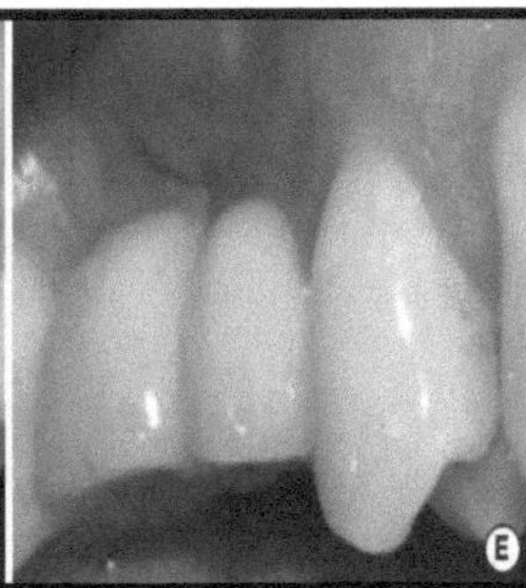

Figure – 11 Clinical views at 12 months postoperatively[97]

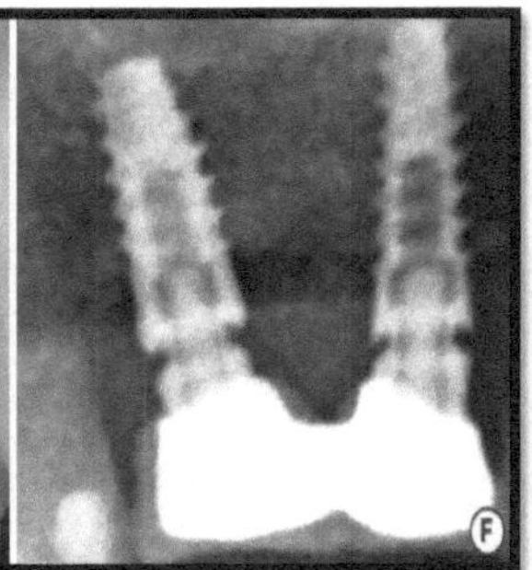

Figure – 12 Defect fill at 12 months postoperatively[97]

Ozonated Therapy in Toothbrush Decontamination

Toothbrushes upon use, rapidly become contaminated by a plethora of oral microorganisms including bacteria, viruses and fungi. Bacteria isolated from conventional brushes showed increasing rates when compared to antibacterial ozonated water used brushes by the same individuals.[99-100]

Method

Sampling preparation –

Volunteers were asked to bring their brushes to the laboratory in plastic sterilized bags.The bristles from each brush were aseptically trimmed off and transferred into a tube with 9 ml sterile phosphate buffered saline (PBS) solution. The content was vigorously vortexed for 3 min in order for the non-strongly adherent cells to be detached.Afterwards, this same content was vigorously shaken in a cold bath for 10 min in order for the sessile cells to be detached. Moreover, serial tenfold dilutions in PBS were prepared for microbiological evaluation.[100]

Microbiological analysis

One hundred microliters from each dilution were plated onto different selective and non-selective growth media as follows: Mannitol salt agar was used to quantitatively detect Staphylococcus sp. Representative colonies were picked and subjected to Gram-stain, catalase and coagulase tests. MacConkey agar was used to enumerate presumptively Enterobacteriaceae. Characteristic colonies appeared within 24 h were confirmed by the IMVC test.[100]

Moreover, the following media were used: MRS agar for the recovery of Lactobacillus, Mitis salivarius agar for total Streptococci and Columbia agar supplemented with blood (5%) for the aerobes and facultative anaerobes. Finally, sabouraud dextrose agar was used for cultivation of yeasts and moulds. Incubation of the plates was performed accordingly to the involved medium aerobically for 24 h at 37 8C or anaerobically for at least 5 days at 37 ^{0}C.[100]

Ozone sanitation trials

The decimal dilutions of our samples (T: 20 8C) were ozone saturated by using a commercial ozone gas generator through a sterilized micro-diffuser and samples for microbiological analysis were drawn after 5, 10, 15, 20 and 30 min. 100 ml from the ozonated suspensions were plated on all previous growth media and incubated accordingly. A quantiative evaluation of the microbial growth achieved by inoculation of 10^{-1} to 10^{-7} dilutions from each sample onto Columbia blood agar. Ozone concentrations were estimated photometricaly with the indigo method by using a commercially available kit. Final ozone concentration succeeded is reported to 3– 3.5 ppm.[100]

A quantitative evaluation of the microbial growth was achieved after the end of the ozonation. The re-growth profile of bacteria was estimated by total counting of the recovered bacteria (CFU/ml). Count of microorganisms isolated per brush varied between 102 and 107 CFU. Candida albicans was present in used toothbrushes.[100]

No obligate anaerobes were isolated. Members of Streptococcaceae family were regularly found (65.2%) belonging to the following species: Streptococcus pyogenes, S. mutans, S. mitis, S. oralis, S. sobrinus, S. viridans, S. salivarius, S. sanguis, Aerococcus viridans. A. viridans and S. mutans were more frequently isolated on children's toothbrushes while Staphylococcus aureus and S. epidermidis were found on adult brushes. Escherichia coli, Pseudomonas sp. and Enterococcus sp., were also recovered. We found that the ozone treatment decreased gradually the microbial load.However, a bacterial regrowth was effective following short ozonation period. Decontamination was complete after an extended exposure to ozone for 30 min.[100]

Ozone Toxicity:

Complications caused by ozone therapy are infrequent at 0.0007 per application[101].

Known side-effects are:[101]

1. **Epiphora**
2. **Upper respiratory irritation**
3. **Rhinitis**
4. **Cough**
5. **Headache**
6. **Occasional nausea, vomiting**
7. **Shortness of breath**
8. **Blood vessel swelling**
9. **Poor circulation**
10. **Heart problems**

European cooperation of Medical Ozone Societies prohibited the intravenous injections of Ozone gas due to risk of air embolism.[4]

In the event of an ozone intoxication the patient must be placed in the supine position, inhale humid oxygen, and take ascorbic acid, vitamin E, and n-acetylcysteine. Because of ozone's highly oxidative power, all materials that come in contact with the gas must be ozone resistant, such as glass, silicon, and Teflon.[102]

Conclusion

Conclusion

The use of ozone has opened new vistas in treatment modalities. Ozone has a variety of beneficial effects, including as immunostimulant, analgesic, anti-hypoxic, detoxicating, antibacterial, bioenergetic and biosynthetic effects. It is the prefect therapy option for paediatric children due to easy, faster, minimally invasive and completely painless and atraumatic character, which increases patient acceptability and compliance. Dental treatment in children is frequently complex and ozone could support the doctor to improving the approach and prognosis with young children, non-cooperative and for special health care need children. Ozone therapy presents great advantages when used as support for following treatment including oral prophylaxis, prevention of caries, remineralization of pit and fissure caries, remineralization of root and smooth surface caries, cavity disinfection and restoration, desensitization of extremely sensitive tooth, endodontic treat such as obturation, irrigation of canal with ozonated water, orthodontics patients, oral surgeries, soft tissue pathoses, tooth brush decontamination and implantology.

References

References

1. Makkar S, Makkar M. Ozone-treating dental infections. Indian J Stomatol. 2011;2 (4):256-59.
2. Amario M, Carlo C, Natale S M, Memè L, Marzo G. Application of Ozone therapy in Paediatric Dentistry. Appl Sci. 2022;12(21):1-11.
3. Nogales C G, Ferrari P A, Kantorovich EO, LageMarques JL. Ozone Therapy in Medicine and Dentistry. J Contemp Dent Pract. 2008;4(9):75-84.
4. Garg R, Tandon S. Ozone: A new face of dentistry. J Dent Sci. 2009;7(2):23-27
5. Seidler V, Linetskiy I, Hubalkova H, Stankova H, Smucler R, Mazanek J. Ozone and its usage in General Medicine and Dentistry. Prague Medical Report. 2008; 10(9):5-13.
6. Saha S, Soni K, Pandey P, Saha S Ozone in pediatric dentistry. A miracle therapy. I D A. 2018;34(2):6-9.
7. Rudrakshi C1, Prabhuji M L V. Ozone therapy in dentistry. J Ind Dent Assoc. 2014;8(9):15-22.
8. Ebensberger U, Pohl Y, Filippi A. PCNA-expression of cementoblasts and fibroblasts on the root surface after extraoral rinsing for decontamination. Dent Traum. 2002;18(50:262-6.
9. Murakami H, Mizuguchi M, Hattori M, Ito Y, Kawai T, Hasegawa J. Effect of denture cleaner using ozone against methicillin-resistant Staphylococcus aureus and E. coli T1 phage. Dent Mater J. 2002;21(1):53–60.
10. Nagayoshi M, Fukuizumi T, Kitamura C, Yano J, Terashita M, Nishihara T. Efficacy of ozone on survival and permeability of oral microorganisms. Oral Microbiol Immunol. 2004;19(4):240-6.

11. Nagayoshi M, Kitamura C, Fukuizumi T, Nishihara T, Terashita M. Antimicrobial effect of ozonated water on bacteria invading dentinal tubules. J Endod. 2004;30(11):778-81.

12. Hems RS, Gulabivala K, Ng YL, Ready D, Spratt DA. An in vitro evaluation of the ability of ozone to kill a strain of Enterococcus faecalis. Int Endod J. 2005;38(1):22-9.

13. Huth KC, Jakob FM, Saugel B, Cappello C, Paschos E, Hollweck R, et al. Effect of ozone on oral cells compared with established antimicrobials. Eur J Oral Sci. 2006;114(5):435–40.

14. Estrela C, Estrela CR, Decurcio Dde A, Silva JA, Bammann LL. Antimicrobial potential of ozone in an ultrasonic cleaning system against Staphylococcus aureus. Braz J. 2006;17(2):134–8.

15. Polydorou OPK, Hahn P. Antibacterial effect of an ozone device and it1s comparison with two dentin-bonding systems. Eur Jo Oral Sci. 2006;114(4):349–53.

16. Celiberti P, Pazera P, Lussi A. The impact of ozone treatment on enamel physical properties. Am J Dent. 2006;19(1):67–72.

17. Muller P, Guggenheim B, Schmidlin PR. Efficacy of gasiform ozone and photodynamic therapy on a multispecies oral biofilm in vitro. Eur J Oral Sci. 2007;115(1):77–80.

18. Kshitish, D. & Laxman, V. K. The use of ozonated water and 0.2% chlorhexidine in the treatment of periodontitis patients: A clinical and microbiologic study. Indian J Dent Res. 2010;21(3):341-8.

19. Skurska, A.; Pietruska, M. D.; Paniczko-Drezek, A.; Dolinska, E.; Zelazowska-Rutkowska, B.; Zak, J.; et al. Evaluation of the influence of ozonotherapy on the

clinical parameters and MMP levels in patients with chronic and aggressive periodontitis. Adv Med Sci. 2010;55(2):297-07.

20. Dhingra, K. & Vandana, K. L. Management of gingival inflammation in orthodontic patients with ozonated water irrigation: a pilot study. Int J Dent Hyg. 2011;9(4):296-02.

21. El Hadary, A. A.; Yassin, H. H.; Mekhemer, S. T.; Holmes, J. C. & Grootveld, M. Evaluation of the effect of ozonated plant oils on the quality of osseointegration of dental implants under the influence of Cyclosporin A. An in vivo study. J Oral Implantol. 2011;37(2):247-57.

22. Huth, K. C.; Quirling, M.; Lenzke, S.; Paschos, E.; Kamereck, K.; Brand, K.; et al. Effectiveness of ozone against periodontal pathogenic microorganisms. J Oral Sci. 2011;119(3):204-10.

23. Hauser-Gerspach, I.; Vadaszan, J.; Deronjic, I.; Gass, C.; Meyer, J.; Dard, M.; et al. Influence of gaseous ozone in peri-implantitis: bactericidal efficacy and cellular response. An in vitro study using titanium and zirconia. Clin Oral Investig. 2012;16(4):1049-59.

24. Kronenberg, O.; Lussi, A. & Ruf, S. Preventive effect of ozone on the development white spot lesions during multibracket appliance therapy. Angle Orthodot. 2009;79(1):64-9.

25. Chandra. S.P, Chandrasekhar.R, Uloopi. K.S. Success of root filling with zinc-oxide ozonated oil in primary molars. Eur Arch Peaditar Dent. 201418(2):111-15.

26. Beretta. M, Canova. F A new method for deep caries treatment in primary teeth using ozone: a retrospective study. Eur J Pediatr.2017;18(2)111-15.

27. Kucuk. F, Yildirum. S, Cetiner.S Cytotoxicity assessment of diferent doses of ozonated water on dental pulp cells. Oral Health. 2021;21(32)1-7.

28. Luppieri V, Manfra A, Ronfani L, Chermetz M, Cadenaro M. Ozone Therapy for Early Childhood Caries (ECC) Treatment: An In Vivo Prospective Study. Appl Sci. 2022;12(4):1-10.

29. Hamid M Y, Deleme H Z, Khudhur S J. Histological Assessment of the Oral Soft Tissue Regenerative Capacity of Hyaluronic Acid and Ozonated Oil. An in vitro study. Al-Rafidain Dent J. 2023;23(1):158-68.

30. Ximenes, Cardoso M, Astorga M, Arnold F, Pimenta R. Antimicrobial activity of ozone and NaF- chlorhexidine on early childhood caries. Braz Oral Res. 2017; 31(5):1-10.

31. Seidler V, Linetskiy I, Hubalkova H, Stankova H, Smucler R, Mazanek J. Ozone and its usage in General Medicine and Dentistry. Prague Medical Report. 2008;109(1):5-13.

32. Malik. T, Kaura1. S, Kakria. P Dental Ozone: A Boon for Dentistry. Indian J Dent Sci. 2020;12(1):49-52.

33. Agrillo A, Sassano P, Rinna C, Priore P, Iannetti G. Ozone therapy in extractive surgery on patients treated with bisphosphonates. J Craniofac Surg. 2007; 18(5):1068-70.

34. Saini R. Ozone therapy in dentistry: A strategic review. J Nat Sc Biol Med. 2011;2(2):151-3.

35. Karapetian VE, Lowden E and Zöller JE. The Use of Ozone in Periimplantitis-Treatment - Das Deutsche Zahnärzteblatt. 2007;116(5):214-18.

36. Gupta. M, Abhishek. Ozone: An emerging prospect in dentistry. In J Den Sci. 2012;1(4):47-50.

37. Eregowda NI, Parameswarappa P. Ozone in dentistry. Indian J Dent Adv. 2015;7(1):36-40.

38. Tapia AS, Talbott B. Ozone in Preeclampsia of pregnancy. Case report. Revista Española de Ozonoterapia. 2018;8(1):99-108.

39. Calabrese EJ, Kojola WH, Carnow BW. Ozone: A possible cause of hemolytic anemia in glucose-6-phosphate dehydrogenase deficient individuals. J Toxicol Environ Health. 1977;2(3):709-12.

40. Huffman LJ, Judy DJ, Brumbaugh K, Frazer DG, Reynolds JS, McKinney WG, et al. Hyperthyroidism increases the risk of ozone-induced lung toxicity in rats. Toxicol Appl Pharmacol. 2001;173(10:18-26.

41. Estrela C, Estrela CR, Decurcio DdA, Silva JA, Bammann LL. Antimicrobial potential of ozone in an ultrasonic cleaning system against Staphylococcus aureus. Braz Dent J. 2006;17(2):134-8.

42. Gupta. M et al. Ozone: An emerging prospect in dentistry. In J Den Sci. 2012;1(4):47-50.

43. Malik U, Gulzar A, Sunil MK, Anjali. Ozone Therapy in Dentistry. J Dent. 2018;5(3):17-19.

44. Tyagi A, Khattri S. Periodontal application of ozone therapy. J Acad Dent Educ. 2023;9(2):80-5.

45. Solomon S. Stratospheric ozone depletion: a review of concepts and history. Reviews of Geophysics. 1999;37(3):275-316.

46. Gupta G, Mansi B. Ozone therapy in periodontics. J med life. 2012;5(1):59-67.

47. Saeed NHGH, Fattah CH, Amin KA, Kadir SK. Evaluation of the antimicrobial effects of ozonated water on the sanitization of endodontic files contaminated with C. Albicans. Sulaimani Dent J. 2015;2(2).

48. Mudd, Freeman BA Reaction of Ozone with biological membranes S.D. Lee (Ed.), Biochemical effects of environmental pollutants. 1987;46(2):168-79.

49. Gupta S, Deepa D. Applications of ozone therapy in dentistry. J Oral Res Rev 2016; 8(2):86-91.

50. J.B. Mudd, Freeman BA Reaction of Ozone with biological membranes S.D. Lee (Ed.), Biochemical effects of environmental pollutants

51. Kakran A, Namdev R., Rajput N., Negi S., Kaushik H. Ozone Therapy in dental practice - A concise review. Clinical Dentistry 2022; XVI; 22-29.

52. Shashikiran N, Hadakar S, Gaonkar N, et al. Ozone and Nanotechnology in Dentistry. Cambridge Scholars Publishing, 2022

53. Singh T, Majumdar S, Ghosh AK, et al. Application of Ozone Therapy in Dentistry, A Review. J Adv Med Dent Scie Res. 2014; 2(3): 44-7.

54. Sujatha B, Manoj Kumar MG, Pratap Gowd MJ. Raja Vardhan. Ozone therapy – a paradigm shift in dentistry. An Open Access Peer Reviewed E. J Health Sci. 2013; 2(3):1-10.

55. Schwartz.A, Sanchez.GM, Madrid declarationon ozone therapy.international community of ozozne therapy. 2020;4(3):4-104.

56. Anumula L, Kumar KS, Krishna CM, et al. Antibacterial activity of freshly prepared ozonated water and chlorhexidine on Mutans Streptococcus when used as an oral rinse - A randomised clinical study. J Clin Diagn Res. 2017; 11(7):05–08.

57. Forssten SD, Björklund M and Ouwehand AC. Streptococcus mutans, caries and simulation models. Nutrients. 2010; (3):290–298.

58. Casu. C, Orrù. G, Fais. S, Mazur. M, Grassi. R, Efficacy of ozonated water as a PS in photodynamic therapy: A tool for dental caries management? An in vitro study. J Pub Heal Resh. 2023;12(2):1-8

59. Bjørndal L, Larsen T, Thylstrup A. A clinical and microbiological study of deep carious lesions during stepwise excavation using long treatment intervals. Caries Res. 1997;31(6):411–17.

60. Ricketts DN, Kidd EA, Beighton D. Operative and microbiological validation of visual, radiographic and electronic diagnosis of occlusal caries in non-cavitated teeth judged to be in need of operative care. Br Dent J. 1995;179(6):214–20.

61. Sancakli HS, Siso SH, Yildiz SO, Gökçe YB. Antibacterial effect of surface pretreatment techniques against Streptococcus mutans. Niger J Clin Pract.2018;21(2):170-175.

62. Weerheijm KL, Kreulen CM, de Soet JJ, Groen HJ, van Amerongen WE. Bacterial counts in carious dentine under restorations: 2-year in vivo effects. Caries Res. 1999;3(3):130–34.

63. Almaz ME, Sönmez IŞ. Ozone therapy in the management and prevention of caries. J Formos Med Assoc 2015;1(3):3-11

64. Baysan A, Whiley RA, Lynch E. Antimicrobial effect of a novel ozone-generating device on micro-organisms associated with primary root carious lesions in vitro. Caries Res. 2000;34(6):498–01.

65. Gokcen EY, Oz FT, Ozcelik B, Orhan AI, Ozgul BM. Assessment of antibacterial activity of different treatment modalities in deciduous teeth: an in vitro study Biotechnol Biotechnol Equip. 2016;30(8):1192-08.

66. Beretta. M,Federici.Canova. A new method for deep caries treatment in primary teeth using ozone: a retrospective study. Eup J Pediatric Dent. 2017;18(2):111-15

67. Olivi R, Olivi F. Odontoiatria Infantile Pratica. Edizioni Martina: Bologna; 2007.

68. Lynch E. Ozone: the revolution in dentistry. Quintessence: Copenhagen, Chicago; 2004.

69. Baysan A, Lynch E. The use of ozone in dentistry and medicine. Part 2. Ozone and root caries. Prim Dent Care J Fac Gen Dent Pract. 2006;13(7):37–41.

70. Samuel SR, Dorai S, Khatri SG, Patil ST. Effect of ozone to remineralize initial enamel caries: in situ study. Clin Oral Investig .2016:20(11):1109–13.

71. Sobral, M. A. P. & Garone Netto, N. Clinical aspects about the etiology of cervical dentin hypersensitivity. Revista de Odontologia da Universidade de São Paul. 1999;13(2):189-95.

72. Brännström, M. & Garberoglio, R. Occlusion o dentinal tubules under superficial attrited dentine. Swed DenT J. 1980;4(3):87-91.

73. Moretzsohn, M. & Campos, I. Hipersensibilidade dentinária: Ainda um problema? Revista Brasileira de Odontologia.2001 Mastrantonio, S. S. & Ramalho, L. T. O. Mouse connective tissue reaction to polyurethane derived from castor oil. Revista de. Odontologia da. 2003;32(1):31-37.

74. Mastrantonio, S. S. & Ramalho, L. T. O. (2003). Mouse connective tissue reaction to polyurethane derived from castor oil. Revista de. Odontologia da. 2010;32(1):31-37.

75. Goldberg, M., Kulkarni, A.B., Young, M. & Boskey, A. Dentin: structure, composition and mineralization. Frontiersin Bioscience. 2011;3(1):711-35.

76. Veena H. R., Afigith Mathew C., Daniel R. A., Shubha P., Sreeparvathy R. & Pradhan N. An in vitro analysis of the effect of adjunctive use of ozonated oil with a desensitizing agent on dentinal tubule occlusion. Journal of Oral Biology Craniofacial Research. 2022;10(4):727-732.

77. Souza. WSS, Silveira. GNT, Oliveira. HDSF, Glória. JCR, Gonçalves. PF. Dentin hypersensitivity treatment with ozonated oil: a randomized controlled tripleblind clinical trial. Resh Soc And Dev. 2021;10(17):1-10.

78. Morrow D, Wood DP, Speechley M. Clinical effect of subgingival chlorhexidine irrigation on gingivitis in adolescent orthodontic patients. Am J Orthod Dentofac Orthop. 1992;101(5):408-13.

79. Weinstein E, Khurana H, Mandel ID. Lactate dehydrogenase isoenzymes in gingival fluid. Arch Oral Biol. 1972;17(7):375–76.

80. Lamster IB, Mandella RD, Gordon JM. Lactate dehydrogenase activity in gingival crevicular fluid collected with filter paper strips: analysis in subjects with non-inflamed and mildly inflamed gingiva. J Clin Periodontol. 1985; 12(7): 153–161.

81. Kishinda M, Sato S, Ito K. Comparison of the effect of various periodontal rotary instruments on the surface characterstics of root surface. J Oral Sci. 2004;4(6):1-8.

82. Annie. V, Mathew. JJ, Ambooken. M, Kachappilly. AJ, JOHNY.T. Management of Chronic Periodontitis Using Subgingival Irrigation of Ozonized Water: A Clinical and Microbiological Study. J Clin Diag Resh. 2015;9(8):89-93.

83. Baysan A, Lynch E. Clinical reversal of the root caries using ozone. Am J Dent. 2007;20(4):203-08.

84. Baysan A, Lynch E. The use of ozone in dentistry and medicine. Prim Dent Care. 2005;12(7):47-52.

85. Lynch E. Evidence – based caries reversal using ozone. J Esthet Restor Dent. 2008;20(15):218-22.

86. Kazancioglu. H. O, Kurklu. E, Ezirganli. S. Effects of ozone therapy on pain, swelling, and trismus following third molar surgery. Int J Oral Maxillofac Surg. 2014;43(4):644-48.

87. Trairatvorakul. C, Chunlasikaiwan S. Success of pulpectomy with zinc oxide eugenol vs calicium hydroxide/Iodoform paste in primary molars: A clinical study. Pediatr Dent. 2008;30(19):303-08.

88. Tronstad. L. Recent development in endodontics research. J Dent Res. 1995;16(9):161-71.

89. Goerig. AC, Camp JH. Root canal treatment in primary teeth. Pediatr Dent. 1983;5(3):33-37.

90. Chawla HS, Mani SA, Tewari A, Goyal A. Calcium hydroxide as a root canal treatment in primary teeth- A piolet study. J Indian Soc Pedo Prev Dent. 1985;7(3):123-9.

91. Guinesi. AS,Filho IB et al. Ozonized oils -A qualitative and quanditative analysis. Braz Dent J. 2011;22(7):37-40.

92. Lindhe J, Meyle J; Group D of European Workshop on Periodontology. Peri-implant diseases: consensus report of the sixth European Workshop on Periodontology. J. Clin. Periodontol. 2008;35(3):282-85.

93. Lang NP, Berglundh T; Working Group 4 of Seventh European Workshop on Periodontology. Periimplant diseases: where are we now consensus of the Seventh European Workshop on Periodontology. J Clin Periodontol. 2011;38(10):78-81.

94. Mombelli A, Lang NP. Microbial aspects of implant dentistry. J. Periodontol. 2000;4(2):74-80.

95. Esposito M, Grusovin MG, Worthington HV. Interventions for replacing missing teeth: treatment of periimplantitis. Cochrane Database Syst Rev. 2012:18(1):1-8

96. McKenna DF, Borzabadi-Farahani A, Lynch E. The effect of subgingival ozone and/or hydrogen peroxide on the development of peri-implant mucositis: a double-blind randomized controlled trial. Int J Oral Maxillofac Implants. 2013;28(6):1483-9.

97. Isler. SC, Unsal. B, Soysal. F,Ozcan. G, Peker. E. et al. The effects of ozone therapy as an adjunct to the surgical treatment of peri- implantitis. J Periodontal Implant Sci. 2018;48(3):136-51.

98. Sammons RL, Kaur D, Neal P. Bacterial survival and biofilm formation on conventional and antibacterial toothbrushes. Biofilms .2004;10(2):123–30.

99. Haffajee AD, Smith C, Torresyap G, Thompson M, Guerrero D, Socransky SS. Efficacy of manual and powered toothbrushes II. Effect on microbiological parameters. J Clin Periodontolo. 2001;28(10):947–54.

100. Bezirtzoglou. E, Cretoiu. SM, Moldoveanu. M,Alexopoulos.A , Lazar.V. A quantitative approach to the effectiveness of ozone against microbiota organisms colonizing toothbrushes. J Dent. 2008;36(8):600-05.

101. Naik. SV, Rajeshwari. K, Kohli. S, Zohabhasan. S, Bhatia. S Ozone- A Biological Therapy in Dentistry- Reality or Myth J Open Dent. 2016;11(10):196-06.

102. Pattanaik B, Jetwa D, Pattanaik S, Manglekar S, Naitan DN, Dani A. Ozone therapy. J Interdisciplin. Dent. 2011;1(2):87-92.

65

Kolibri 360 GmbH
Ferdinand-Jühlke-Straße 7
99095 Erfurt, Deutschland
produktsicherheit@kolibri360.de

Druck:
CPI Druckdienstleistungen GmbH
im Auftrag der
Kolibri 360 GmbH
Ferdinand-Jühlke-Str. 7
99095 Erfurt